Your First Marathon

A Beginners Guide To Marathon Training, Marathon Preparation and Completing Your First Marathon

Richard Bond

DEDICATION

For Louise, my extraordinary partner who's support and encouragement has helped me accomplish all that I have today. I love you very much.

CONTENTS

Intentionally Left Blank

INTRODUCTION

Running your first marathon is a daunting task. There are so many things to think about before you even start such as, what race to enter, which training program should you follow, should you eat differently, what equipment or technology can help, are you physically and mentally strong enough to complete it and the list goes on. This book will help you answer all of these questions and allieviate some of the fear attached to running a marathon for the first time.

What are you going to learn?

I'm going to help you select the appropriate race for your needs. I'm going to show you how to train depending on your goals – whether it's to get you over the finish line, or complete a marathon in under 4 hours. I'm going to teach you the mindset to have to be successful. I'll show you the equipment and gadgets that can help you cross the finish line. I'll teach you the basics on nutrition and hydration. I'll show you how to prepare for a race. How to avoid/minimise injuries and how to recover. I'll teach you how to avoid mistakes and share the top tips that helpd me cross the line for the first time.

This book is designed to help the first time marathon runner cross the finish line in a simple and effective way.

Are you ready to take on one of the biggest challenges of your life?

THE MARATHON: AN INTRODUCTION

Legend has it that in the year 490 BC, an Athenian soldier named Pheidippides ran from the town of Marathon, Greece to Athens, a distance of about 26 miles, to announce that the Greeks have been victorious over the invading Persians. Pheidippides ran non-stop the whole way that when he arrived in Athens to pronounce the great news, he only managed to exclaim "Victory!" before collapsing to his death.

Fast-forward to 1896 and the marathon became one of the first Olympic sports in the very first running of the Olympics. At that time, the race was only pegged at 40 kilometers, and only 17 runners lined up at the starting line to compete in the first ever Olympic marathon. Out of those 17 valiant competitors, only 8 runners crossed the finish line. The winning time was just a hair under 3 hours by a guy named Spyridon Louis who wore leather shoes donated by his fellow villagers. Fast-forward again another 118 years.

In 2014, 50,869 runners towed the starting line at the New York Marathon. An astounding 50,266 runners managed to cross the finish line. But New York is hardly alone in luring in runners to run the marathon.

Below is a table of the five largest marathon races in history as sorted by venue.

Marathon	Date	Number of Finishers
New York City	11/2/2014	50,564
Chicago	10/12/2014	40,802
Paris	4/07/2013	38,690
London	4/22/2012	36,672
Boston	4/15/1996	35,868

So why do millions of people every year decide to run marathons? Just what is in those 26.2 miles that people are itching to sign up for races, commit the time to train for several weeks, and invest a significant amount of money? Is it the medal? Is it the venue? Is it the idea of having ran a marathon? Is it for health? Or is it for a personal sense of accomplishment?

Your Goals and Motivation for Running a Marathon

Everyone has his or her own reasons for wanting to finish a marathon. Many of the above reasons qualify and there are many others that are not as publicized but are just as meaningful. Of course, there is no "right" or "wrong" reason to run a marathon. Every reason is valid as long as it gets you from mile 0 to mile 26 in one piece. What's more important to remember is your reason for deciding to run in the first place, and to use that reason to fuel your motivation to train and finish on race day.

Let's face it, running a marathon is not easy. It is one of the most challenging tasks you can ever take up, and also one of the most rewarding.

You will often hear this from many speakers who are encouraging you to run your first marathon: less than 0.1% of all the people in the world have completed one. Simply finishing gives you access to one of the most elite clubs in the world. Since when have you ever been a part of top 99.99% of the whole human race?

But that's just the glamor part of it; the mental part is just as rewarding. Running a marathon and the process of training to finish one will tell you a lot about yourself. It will reveal your character. It will show you your weaknesses and force you to overcome those.

So think about your goals and motivation of running a marathon. Is it just to finish one, or do you want to beat a specific time, say 4 hours?

Whatever those goals are, allow those goals to drive and motivate you. Today, as you begin your marathon journey, write those goals on a piece of paper and tape it to your mirror or refrigerator. Look at those goals every day. Remind yourself to always go back to the goal. Because the going will get tough at some point; but if you allow your goals to drive you, and you know why you're out running when you should be somewhere else, you've already won half of the battle.

So this is mile 0… Now, let's get you to mile 26.

HOW TO GET STARTED ON YOUR MARATHON JOURNEY

In the most literal sense, your marathon journey started the very minute you made the decision to run your first marathon. Right then and there, everything changes for you.

The moment you take up that commitment to lace up for a 26 mile race, you can immediately feel the weird mix of excitement and dread that comes with deciding to train for a marathon.

This book is specifically written so from that moment onwards, you feel more excitement and less dread.

The fear of the unknown is one of the most difficult things to overcome for anyone, and the months preceding a marathon can be fraught with challenges that you need to overcome in order to be successful on race day.

Well, do not worry. That's what this book is for.

So, how can you get started? Well, the first thing that you need to do is to pick a race to sign up for. You can't make the decision to complete your first marathon and then kick the can down the road by postponing registration to any race.

Which race should you pick? There are many schools of thought here. One way is to pick a low profile race with a relatively low number of participants. Low profile races can help ease the pressure that is common in big races. There are fewer runners on the road so you do not have to jockey for position. There's not a lot of fanfare so you don't get suckered into running really fast out of the gate.

The downside to low-profile races is that they tend to lack the energy that can help push you on when you're struggling at 18 miles. Inexperienced organizers can lead to serious problems like insufficient hydration stations or complicated race kit claiming.

Aside from the race profile itself, there are also many other considerations for choosing your first race. How's the weather going to be on race day? This is especially important if you are picking a destination race that allows you to travel, but also forces you to run in conditions that are vastly different from your training runs. Even the course profile can be a factor; if you don't scout your races properly, you could end up running on a hilly course when all your training was done on flatter roads.

And as far as destination races go, the excitement of traveling can be a great source of motivation but it can also cause a lot of stress. You have to find the right hotel that's close to the starting line, you have to be familiar with the commuting options at your destination, and you can even be distracted by all the sight-seeing that you plan to do before or after the marathon.

The short answer to selecting the right first marathon is that there is no formula that works for everyone. What's important, however, is that you put the right amount of effort in selecting the race that's perfect for your needs.

Ask yourself these questions:

Do you prefer running in the cold or when it is hot? This can already help you narrow down your options in terms of location and time of the year.

Do you want a race that starts very early in the morning or later in the day? This will help you match your training routine accordingly.

Do you want a hilly or a flatter course? A hilly course isn't always a bad thing if you trained for it, but it can definitely add more challenge into an otherwise already challenging task.

Do you want to travel or stay within the vicinity? Evaluate which one is best according to your situation and decide based on that. You can always travel for your second marathon when you've already established a routine that works.

Would you prefer running in a big or small race? There is some degree of prestige when you complete the New York marathon but not every runner likes to be in a big crowd. Which type of runner are you? Match your race to your preference; and again, you can always go big or small for your next race.

Does your preferred marathon have a cut-off time? Many marathons have a cut-off time of 6 hours which means not finishing within that period will already disqualify you from the race. If you can run fast enough to beat that time, it's well and good; if that, and you just want to finish your first, you might want to consider races that have longer cut-off times to give you more room to work with on race day.

Remember: picking the right race is very important to ensuring your first marathon success. Spend some time thinking about it so you can be sure that you are choosing the best race that will guarantee the least amount of stress with the highest likelihood of success.

Selecting the right training program

Now that you have picked a race, let's get to the meat-and-potatoes of marathon running.

If you want to run a marathon, the most important thing you have to remember is that not everything happens on race day. Your training is the biggest factor that can make or break your race. For the elites, a marathon cannot be won in training, but they can definitely lose it long before they stand on the starting line.

As such, selecting the appropriate training plan cannot be overstated. If you pick the wrong training plan, you're likely to suffer on race day. The wrong training plan can lead to all sorts of problems including higher risk for injury, or peaking too soon and leaving you depleted on race day, or even under-training you for what lies ahead.

To pick the right training plan, the first question to ask is this: what is your goal on your first marathon?

If you are the competitive type, finishing a marathon in under 4 hours is a very doable goal. Just take note that the training demands for that are vastly different from the training demands of just finishing a marathon.

In addition, the level of fitness required going into the training is also significantly different. If you just want to finish a marathon, you can use the training plan we attached here with little to no running experience prior – perhaps completing a 10-km race (6 miles) should be sufficient just to get you into the mindset of being a runner, but it isn't a prerequisite.

To finish a marathon in less than 4 hours, you should ideally be a runner for a couple of years, have completed a half marathon, or be extremely determined and competitive. Consider that you'll need to be able to complete a sub-2 hour half marathon to stand a chance of a 4 hour marathon. So use this as guide to determine if you can finish a marathon in less than 4 hours or if you're the type who just wants to finish a marathon and leave all that competitive stuff for your second go.

Your Marathon Training Plan with the Goal to Finish

Here's the training plan if you just want to finish your first marathon.

Week	Mon	Tue	Wed	Thu	Fri	Sat	Sun
1	Rest	40 mins walk	Rest	40 mins walk	Rest	45 mins walk	Rest
2	Rest	40 mins walk	Rest	40 mins walk	Rest	45 mins walk	Rest
3	Rest	40 mins easy	Rest	40 mins easy	Rest	Long run (50 mins)	Rest
4	Rest	40 mins easy	Rest	40 mins easy	Rest	Rest	Long run (55 mins)
5	Rest	45 mins easy	Rest	45 mins easy	Rest	Long run (60 mins)	Rest
6	Rest	45 mins easy	Rest	45 mins easy	Rest	Long run (70 mins)	Rest
7	Rest	45 mins easy	Rest	45 mins easy	Rest	Rest	Long run (80 mins)
8	Rest	45 mins easy	Rest	45 mins easy	Rest	Rest	Long run (90 mins)
9	Rest	45 mins easy	Rest	45 mins easy	Rest	Long run (105 mins)	Rest
10	Rest	45 mins easy	Rest	45 mins easy	Rest	Rest	Long run (120 mins)
11	Rest	45 mins easy	Rest	45 mins easy	Rest	Rest	Long run (140 mins)
12	Rest	45 mins easy	Rest	45 mins easy	Rest	Long run (75 mins)	Rest

Week	Mon	Tue	Wed	Thu	Fri	Sat	Sun
13	Rest	45 mins easy	Rest	45 mins easy	Rest	Long run (160 mins)	Rest
14	Rest	45 mins easy	Rest	45 mins easy	Rest	Rest	Long run (90 mins)
15	Rest	45 mins easy	Rest	45 mins easy	Rest	Rest	Long run (195 mins)
16	Rest	45 mins easy	Rest	45 mins easy	Rest	Rest	Long run (90mins)
17	Rest	45 mins easy	Rest	45 mins easy	Rest	Rest	Long run (120 mins)
18	Rest	45 mins easy	Rest	45 mins easy	Rest	Rest	Long run (75 mins)
19	Rest	45 mins easy	Rest	45 mins easy	Rest	Long run (210 mins)	Rest
20	Rest	45 mins easy	Rest	45 mins easy	Rest	Rest	Long run (90 mins)
21	Rest	45 mins easy	Rest	45 mins easy	Rest	Long run (60 mins)	Rest
22	45 mins easy	Rest	45 mins easy	Rest	Rest	Rest	Race Day (26.2 miles)

There are some features to this plan that you need to look at in more detail.

First, this is a classic 3 runs/week plan specifically designed for beginners to be as easy as possible without compromising the end-goal of finishing the race. Of course, you can always do more – provided you do not over-train and end up injured – but the plan calls for these runs as a minimum. Most people should be able to do this without any problems.

Second, the first two weeks is basically a walking routine. For people who have a zero running base, this is perfect. It eliminates the reason that people often use to dismiss the idea of running a marathon: they say, "I have no prior running experience." This plan tells you that you don't need one if all that you want to do is finish the marathon.

Third, the foundation of this program is the long run. As we will discuss later on, the long run is a very important component of marathon training. You can miss some of the weekday runs and get by on the program, but always find time to do the prescribed long run within the prescribed week, it's crucial to your success.

Your Sub-4 Hour Marathon Training Plan

Here's the training plan if you want to complete your first marathon in less than 4 hours. The "M" refers to miles of distance that you need to cover in each run.

Week	Mon	Tue	Wed	Thu	Fri	Sat	Sun
1	3M easy	2M steady	4M slow	Rest	Rest	3M easy	7M slow
2	Rest	1M easy, 2M fast, 1M easy	5M slow	2x1.5M fast	Rest	4M easy	8M slow
3	Rest	1M easy, 3M fast, 1M easy	6M slow	3x1M fast	Rest	4M easy	9M slow
4	Rest	1M easy, 2M fast, 1M easy	7M slow	4x800m fast	Rest	4M easy	10km race (sub 50mins)
5	Rest	5M steady	5M slow	6M fartlek	Rest	4M easy	11M slow
6	Rest	1M easy, 3M fast, 1M easy	6M slow	8x400m fast	Rest	4M easy	13M slow
7	Rest	6M steady	7M slow	9x200m hills	Rest	4M easy	15M slow

Week	Mon	Tue	Wed	Thu	Fri	Sat	Sun
8	Rest	1M easy, 2M fast, 1M easy	8M slow	12x60s fast	Rest	3M easy	15M steady (or 13M race)
9	Rest	8M steady	7M slow	12x200m fast	Rest	4M easy	17M slow
10	Rest	1M easy, 3M fast, 1M easy	8M slow	3x1.5M fast	Rest	3M easy	Half marathon (sub 1:50)
11	Rest	10M steady	6M slow	8M fartlek	Rest	5M easy	19M slow
12	Rest	1M easy, 4M fast, 1M easy	7M slow	5x1M fast	Rest	5M easy	22M slow
13	Rest	9M steady	6M slow	6x800m fast	Rest	5M easy	18M slow
14	4M easy	1M easy, 3M fast, 1M easy	5M slow	12x200m hills	Rest	5M easy	12M slow
15	Rest	Rest	4M slow	6x400m fast	Rest	2M easy	RACE DAY!

Unlike the previous training plan, it's worth noting that this one only takes up about 15 weeks of total training. But, a shorter training plan is not a major issue if your fitness base is already established. Besides, you will notice very quickly that this training run requires a higher volume and mileage than the previous plan, and that speaks to the training demand if you want to finish quicker.

Now, without jumping over into the next section of this chapter about all the different runs that you should do in order succeed with your sub-4 hour goal, it is worthwhile to use a couple of quick indicators to assess if this program works for you. You will find those indicators in Week's 4 and 10 of this training plan.

If you want to run a sub-4 marathon, you basically should be fast enough to do a 10-k in less than 50 minutes and a half marathon in about 1 hour and 50 minutes. At this onset, you need to be honest with yourself. If you are far from these finishing times for the indicated distance, I would prescribe that you re-think your goals.

You can always choose to run a marathon with the end-goal of finishing above 4 hours. For that, you'll need an intermediate plan between the two prescribed here. You will find plenty of resources online to help you with your goals.

Alternatively, you can drop your plan to run the marathon in the next few weeks and instead focus on building your fitness to be able to run a sub-50 minute 10-k and a sub 1:50-hour half marathon. Once you have that fitness base in place, you can always come back here and take on the prescribed program.

With your chosen plan in place, let's go ahead and talk about the different types of runs you can do to be successful at completing a marathon.

The different types of run workouts and why you need to do them all

Yes, there are many different types of training runs. For many people, running is one and the same. For marathon training, however, one needs to be more conscious of the different workout types as these can help target different aspects of your training and fitness accordingly.

Long Runs

These are the foundation of every marathon training program. These are designed to get your body ready for the demands of running a marathon lasting several hours. They are also typically done on weekends so you are less likely to be pressured to hurry up and finish.

Another aspect to long runs is that these should almost always been done slower than any other run. The pace of most long runs is often 1-2 minutes/mile slower than your typical running pace. Again, the idea is to allow your body to get used to the idea of running for extended periods.

The last important aspect of long runs is that these need to be done progressively. At the onset of training, your long runs should be in the 60-minutes range. As you build-up fitness, you slowly increase your long run mileage goals. The rule-of-thumb is to increase your mileage by about 10% every week or by 10-15 minutes if you are using a time-based training routine similar to the first plan we included above.

Speedwork

Speedwork, as the name implies, is all about running at a higher pace. In the training plan for completing a marathon, we did not include any speedwork because these aren't necessary. However, if you plan to finish in under-4 hours, speedwork is everything.

The purpose of speedwork is to train your body to run at a higher pace than what you're used to doing.

Most runners are recommended to do speed workouts once a week. The track or treadmill are the best ways to do a speed workout although running on the road can work as well provided you can keep the pace despite all the possible distractions.

To be successful in doing speed workouts, try to adopt segmented repeats where you run a particular distance at 1-2 minutes/mile faster than your typical running pace, and the incorporate short rest breaks per segment. One example is to do 12 x 400-meter track workouts with 1-minute rest periods between each loop. Another example is to do 6 x 800-meter track workouts with 2 mins rest between periods. This will allow you to recover for short periods so you can sustain your target speed longer.

Tempo workouts

Tempo runs are done at speeds slower than a speed workout but faster than your typical run pace. The idea is to sustain the effort at longer distances than what conventional speedwork allows.

For example, if you plan to run a 10-k race in 50 minutes, try running your tempo workouts at 4:45 pace for up to 8 km (5 miles) so you can train your body to hold the effort. The idea behind this workout is to train your body to sustain speed over distance.

Hill repeats

Even in the flattest of marathon courses, the occasional hill pops out when you least expect it and that can be enough to break your morale and turn your legs to mush. This is why hill repeats are important for any serious runner looking to conquer the marathon distance.

Hill repeats work much like speed workouts except that you run up a hill instead of on a flat surface. Adopt the segmented training approach by running up the hill and jogging back down as recovery. 20-50 meters of uphill is plenty and depending on the gradient do 6-10 sets. Try to do hill repeats every 2 weeks or so to help your body adjust to the challenges of running on an incline.

Recovery runs

These are slow runs that are often done within a day of a really hard run. The purpose is to help flush out the lactic acid in your muscles so you can avoid muscle soreness and fatigue. Naturally, these are also short distance runs as you don't want to add any more damage into your legs. A 1-2 mile run at very easy pace would be perfect, say 12 hours after a hard morning run.

These are the basic weapons in your arsenal of training runs that can help you become a more successful runner. If you train smartly and incorporate these into your program, you stand a much better chance of overcoming all 26.2 miles of the marathon and finishing strong in the end.

Other training tips and tricks

You will never run out of tips for the marathon. There will always be something new to learn to help you finish the distance; however, take on too many tips and you'll only end up confused and lost.

To avoid all the confusion, I've compiled the most important tips that helped me during my marathon training.

1. Plan your training. It's not enough that you have a training plan tacked on to the refrigerator. Go one step beyond by scheduling your workouts like you're scheduling a meeting. There are many things in your day that can derail a training run so treat it like any other meeting you must go to and make sure you make time for it regardless of how busy you are.

2. On the days when you skip your training runs, don't try to recover by cramming as much mileage as you can during your next run. Remember: a poorly conceptualized training run is a useless run leading to junk miles. Make sure you understand the purpose of each run – speed, tempo, long run, recovery – and execute accordingly.

3. Don't fall for the "you must run in the morning" trick. Many runners wake up at the unholiest of hours to do their training runs. If you like that, it's great, but there are many others who function better later in the day. The trick is to find the time that suits your body best so you can put in your best effort while on training. Consistency is key in training. There is no right or wrong answer. Make the choice that will increase the chances of you keeping to your program.

4. Use your long runs to practice your nutrition and hydration strategy. Don't wait to try out your new energy gels on race day. Try them during a long run and make sure your body doesn't react negatively to them. The same applies for every piece of running gear that you plan to use on race day. We'll discuss this in more detail in the next chapter.

5. Find time to add strength and core training workouts into your routine. A strong core will help improve your running form and keep you strong throughout the whole race.

6. Don't treat your training like a test and cram in the days leading to the race. You need to taper. The training runs we outlined are designed to allow your body to recover in the last 3 weeks before the big day. Make sure you observe this so you don't show up at

the starting line spent and exhausted.

7. Get enough sleep. If you plan to run early the following morning, make sure you don't schedule anything the night before. Go to bed early so you feel more refreshed for next day's run. Getting the right amount of sleep is as important as the training program and nutrition.

These are just some training tips but these are extremely important. Make sure you incorporate these into your training so you can put yourself in the best position to succeed.

Mental tips for the marathon training

Ask anyone who has finished the marathon and they will tell you one thing: the mental battle in those 26.2 miles is just as grueling – if not even more demanding – than the physical toll.

This is true: the marathon is a mental sport as much as it is a physical challenge.

At some point in your training and even during the race, you will be tested and pushed to the limit. You will question yourself, and you will have doubt. This is when you need to summon all the mental strength you can muster and overcome the negative thoughts.

So, how do you prepare your mind for the marathon?

First, always keep it in mind that the marathon is not easy. Expect the pain to come and beyond that, expect the unexpected. Even the best-laid plans of mice and men can falter under an out-of-nowhere cramp or a really bad bonk.

The best way to learn to expect the unexpected is to be diligent in your training. Your training isn't just about preparing your body. It is also about preparing your mind. When you train, you subject yourself to the actual challenges of running so that everything becomes familiar. This will help take away the fear and replace it with the confidence that you've already overcome this in training. What I found reassuring during my first marathon training cycle, was that every 'long run' felt the same as the last one – equally difficult. When I ran 6 miles for the first time it was tough, so was 10 miles and 15 miles. This helped to build my confidence.

Second, do not panic. People begin to doubt when they see that they are off their target pace, and so they try to overcompensate and end up putting themselves in more compromising situations.

If something comes along that you didn't expect, do not get side-tracked. Find a solution as you run and try to deal with it. And always keep your mind on your goal, but always remember to adjust if you need to. No goals are static in a marathon. You can always lose this battle but you can always come back to fight another day, so don't get disheartened by something that is threating to ruin your race.

Third, visualize your goal. Imagine: marathon finisher! A medal around your neck. The cheers of the crowd lifting you up as you cross the finish line. All the training paying off. You might be in pain now but you will be a marathon finisher shortly after, and nothing can take that away from you.

Learn to visualize your goal and keep that in your mind to push you forward. Whenever you start doubting, think of the happy circumstance that awaits at the finish line. Trust me: it will be worth all the pain.

Fourth, plan ahead. Have you checked out how many water stations are there on the course? Where is the hill? Are the final 10-kilometers flat or hilly? What is the expected weather on race day? Planning helps put your mind at ease because you've already considered the likely outcomes.

Fifth, find a running mantra to recite to yourself. My personal favorite: pain is temporary, finishing is forever! By keeping this mantra in mind, you'll find unexpected motivation from within that you didn't think you've ever had.

Sixth, soak up all the distraction. 26 miles is a long distance; you can't expect your mind to survive if you count it down per meter. Instead, take the time to enjoy your surroundings, particularly if it is a destination race. You can also dedicate each kilometer or mile to a loved one or friend. There are creative ways to count down the distance so you don't get absorbed into the monotony of the race. Let your thoughts take you somewhere. It's one of the great pleasures to running.

Seventh, fire up your power song and enjoy its soothing tunes. Running with the music on is always a great way to pass time. If you need extra motivation, your favorite song can always help you get out of the doldrums.

The marathon is a mental game, but you don't have to succumb to all the doubts. Apply these tips in training and during the race and you are more likely to finish in high spirits so you soak in all the glory of your astounding accomplishment.

Remember: pain is temporary, but finishing a marathon is forever!

RUNNING GEAR, NUTRITION AND HYDRATION BASICS, AND INJURY PREVENTION

Training is the most important part of your marathon journey but you should not neglect all the other things that can derail you.

Here are some examples:

- A shoe that hurts your knee or ankle, or one that feels too tight.
- A nagging injury from choosing the wrong shoe that you choose to ignore because it's something that you think will go away.
- A wardrobe malfunction, or worst chaffing in the armpit area.
- A really bad cramp due to poor hydration during a really hot race.

These are really simple issues that can compromise your marathon.

The best way to avoid these issues: know the basics of running gear, nutrition and hydration, and injury prevention that will keep you fit and ready on race day through to the finish line.

Running Gear

Let's start with the most important gear as a runner – your shirt… er, I mean your shoes.

Running Shoes

If you're a minimalist who would like to wish that all shoes are banished from the running scene, then this section is undoubtedly for you. Consider: no other body part gets as much pounding during a run than your feet. Failure to protect your feet from all that pounding is like running into a warzone without as much as a bullet-proof vest.

There's just no way to overstate the importance of running shoes, but – and this is extremely important – picking the wrong shoe is just as bad as not wearing any shoe at all. If you get the wrong shoe, you are only increasing your risk of injury. You might as well forget your marathon dreams if you do that.

So, how do you pick the right running shoe?

Here are a few considerations.

1. **Foot Type and Gait Analysis**.

When you head to a shoe store today, you'll find plenty of classifications for running shoes including neutral, stability, and motion control. These classifications are based on different running gaits and foot types. Flat feet require different running shoes to feet with a higher arch. Runners who pronate or supinate – the terms used to describe the way the ankles roll upon impact – need different types of shoes. Running styles (whether you land with your heel, mid-foot, or forefoot) also require different shoe designs.

The best advice is to head to a local running store. Specialty stores often perform gait analysis for free and then recommend the best shoe models that are right for you. They may cost a little extra in the end but remember that investing in good running shoes is paramount if you want to conquer your marathon dream.

2. **Comfort**.

Don't get caught up in all the marketing hype and all the flamboyant styles that are out in the market today. Comfort remains as one of the most crucial factors in shoe selection, and more so if you plan to run 42-kilomeers (and many hundreds more during training). Always try a shoe on and see how it fits. Make your decision based on comfort and only use style as a secondary factor for shoe selection.

3. **Test Drive**.

One of the best things with running specialty stores is that they have a treadmill where you can test drive your shoe for a few minutes. That's important to determine comfort and fit, something that you cannot do by merely putting on a shoe.

If you choose to order online, find a company that allows you to return and replace your purchase so you can still test a shoe before committing to it for the long haul.

Aside from the shoe selection, there are other things you might want to do to help you in your training.

First, it's always important to have at least two pairs that you can interchange in training. An alternative pair, provided it's the right fit, will allow your feet to adjust so you can strengthen your running muscles by subjecting them to different running conditions and styles in training.

Second, make sure you change your shoes every 300 to 400 miles. Shoe performance degrades over time. A shoe used for 300 miles will not have the same cushion and support than a brand new shoe. By replacing your shoe at the right time, you can help prevent injuries by ensuring maximum comfort and protection for your feet.

Running apparel

Pink, blue, red or black? Before you get lost in all the color options, think of fit first. Does it fit properly?

If it's too loose, it will be a distraction while you run. If it's too constricting, it will hinder your breathing, and that's not something that you want while running a marathon.

Your next consideration is the material or fabric used. Nowadays, synthetic fabrics from big and small brand names alike make it possible for shirts to be light while still quickly absorbing sweat. These fabrics are great for running because they take the sweat off of your body quickly without making your running clothes heavy or soggy.

In colder weather, manufacturers are also now able to supply a wide array of warmers and thermals that remain light while still insulating you from the cold. This would be great if you plan to run a marathon in the fall which is common marathon season for many countries around the world.

You might also want to consider using compression apparel. There is still some debate as the effectiveness of these types of clothing in enhancing performance and delaying the onset of cramps. Some swear by them while others say they don't work. Either way, compression apparel can be a personal choice and you should find time to try at least one compression shorts or tights to see if they work for you.

If not, you can also have the option of using compression socks or calf sleeves while still wearing traditional running shorts. This is often a great solution for many runners who feel that compression shorts are much too revealing but would still want the benefit of using compression apparel.

Lastly, you should also consider wearing a running visor or cap depending on the weather. In hot weather, a visor might be preferable to allow your head to still vent out the heat while protecting you from the sun's glare. In colder weather, a running cap might be more preferable than a bonnet so you can insulate your head as you run.

Regardless of your choice of running clothes, the best marathon advice you can get when it comes to running apparel is to never experiment on race day. The rule is to wear in training what you plan to wear on race day.

This will give you time to get comfortable with your choice of clothing, or even give up on some selections in favor of others when there are issues like chafing or wrong fit. Your long runs are the best way to try on the running apparel that you want to wear on race day because these are the runs that closely simulate your actual marathon run.

With so many selections, you are sure to get one that's just right for you.

Gadgets

We can't leave the subject of running gear without touching on the topic of gadgets. In this day and age of technological abundance, you can easily find a lot of gadgets designed to help you track your running metrics. While not everyone is enamored with the idea of sophisticated gadgets "dictating" your running habits, you also cannot deny that having one can be extremely helpful in monitoring your run mileage, pace, and many other important indicators such as your heart rate so you can quantify the intensity of your workouts.

The most popular selection nowadays are running watches from such brands as Garmin, Polar, Timex, and Suunto among others. There are also new players that have recently introduced their own product to the market including Tomtom, Adidas miCoach, and several others.

If you are planning to buy a watch, have a very clear goal in mind as to what it is that you exactly need. Some of these watches with very sophisticated capabilities can also be very expensive. If you are not sure about your running beyond your first marathon, it might be advisable to refrain from buying very expensive running watches and instead choose ones that are in the lower-priced range.

If you don't want to purchase a new running watch, that's perfectly reasonable, and there are other options that can still help you track running performance. Why not try an app on your smartphone instead? For running, apps like Strava, Nike+, Endomondo, and Runtastic are great options that you can download for free so you can use your phone to monitor your running mileage, pace and other indicators.

In the end, buying running gadgets is entirely up to you. If you plan to continue running for a long time, investing in a good running watch can be a very worthwhile expense. The important thing to remember is that you need to know your goals and adapt your spending accordingly.

Nutrition and Hydration Basics

With all the training that you will be doing, you need to do your body a favor and nourish it properly like you would put fuel into a high performance car.

Nutrition

Your body needs good healthy carbs in order to fuel your workouts. The best way to get carbs is to eat whole grains like quinoa, brown rice, oatmeal and muesli. You can also add fruits to your diet as these provide a great nutritional balance of healthy carbs, vitamins and minerals. Bananas, for example, contain about 31 grams of carbs while also being rich in potassium which is great for the heart.

So, how should you eat relative to your workout time? Here are some tips.

- **Before a workout.** Always try to eat not less than an hour before your workout time. A full-meal can leave you feeling sluggish and weak. Instead, try eating smaller portions of about 100 calories to fuel your workout. This can be in the form of a bowl of whole-grain cereals or two bananas, or even a morning power shake. If you're running longer, however, try to eat more with added protein into your meal so you can power yourself through to the workout. Peanut butter and bananas work really great for this purpose so you should give it a try.

- **During your training run.** For shorter runs, taking in solid food isn't really necessary. For longer runs, try to pack some energy bars or energy gels and nourish as you go. Everyone differs in the way they consume food but as a rough guide, you should try eating a bar or a gel pack every 40-45 minutes while you're on the road.

- **After your workout.** Try to eat within 30 minutes after your workout. This will allow you to replenish your energy reserves. A popular choice among runners nowadays is milk chocolate for recovery. You should give it a try.

- **General diet.** As a rule, a runner's diet should have about 60% carbs, 20% protein, and 20% fat. This rough distribution of nutrients will allow your body to get its fair share of fuel while still allowing you to maintain weight and stay in shape.

Try to eat healthy when you are training. You don't have to do any type of diet but you should be careful with what you eat. Try eating more fruits and vegetables, nuts and whole grains, and lean meats. This will give you the best chance of balancing nutrition with keeping your weight down so you can be at your best on race day.

Hydration

There is no secret to proper hydration. When you are not working out, the best rule to follow is that the more water you drink, the better it is for your body. During your workout, however, the rules are a bit different.

First, always drink enough that you do not get dehydrated. Dehydration can severely impact performance and even kill at the very worst of cases.

A common rule of thumb is to drink 5-8 ounces (142-227ml) of fluid every 15 minutes while you are working out. If you are running in hot weather or you are the type who perspires more than the average person, you should increase this water intake by a couple of ounces to compensate for the extra fluid loss.

You should also consider drinking sports drinks that are packed with electrolytes to replenish the salts that you are losing during the run. Gatorade is the most popular sports drink out on the market but there are other options that you can try if your body doesn't take to Gatorade well.

As a last note, remember that drinking too much while on the run can be bad too so keep an eye on your fluid intake. Excessively drinking water can lead to a condition known as hypernatremia which occurs when your body's electrolyte concentration goes below a certain threshold.

This happens because you naturally release electrolytes as you perspire. Combine that with excessive water intake and you end up with a lower electrolyte concentration which can impair muscle function and cause other problems. Some runners have died from hypernatremia so it is important to pay attention and not drink too much because you think you have to.

Injury Prevention and Recovery

During training, the last thing that you need is to get injured. So how can you prevent injury while keeping to your training plan?

Listen to your body

It's often tempting to try to do more and ignore all the aches and pains during a run but the truth is, pain is your body's way of telling you that something's wrong and you need to back off. There's no shame in cutting a training run short because you felt something is wrong. It's preferable to be cautious than to pay for it later on.

What you should do at the first sign of pain that only worsens as you run is to stop and take some days off. Instead of running, try light walking, or even cross-training to an activity that has minimal impact to the area that hurts. Cycling on a stationary bike can be a good cross-training activity.

Then, when you resume running, try doing it at a slower pace and about half the distance of your typical runs. This will allow you to assess your body's reactions. If necessary, take additional days off or even schedule an appointment with a sports doctor so you can get to the root of the problem early on before it gets worse.

Do not take rest for granted

This is often true of people who are either too competitive or want to make up for lost mileage. Rest is in your training plan for a purpose. It allows you to heal and recover for the next workout.

When you skip your rest periods, you subject your body to a higher risk of injury because it is fatigued and likely weak. So make sure you respect your planned rest periods and give your body a break so it can repair itself for the next set of training runs.

Add strength-training into your program

Injury is often caused by a compensating body part. This happens when one part is weaker than the other and the stronger part is forced to carry more load than necessary. Over time, this can lead to serious injuries that suddenly flare up without warning.

Strength-training helps address this by promoting balance. Balance eliminates areas of weaknesses so you avoid forcing a body part to compensate. This is where a healthy dose of core, leg, and back workouts will do wonders for your running.

I recommend adding 1 to 2 strength workouts a week to compliment your running.

Memorize this: R.I.C.E.

RICE is code for Rest, Ice, Compression, and Elevation. Experienced runners know this by heart. After each workout, give your muscles some much-needed TLC by resting and icing your legs to help flush out the lactic acid, then adding compression, and elevating your legs while you sleep. This method to help ease soreness and recovery.

Get a massage

After all the work you did, a little massage can be a great tool to reward yourself and also to help loosen your tired and tensed muscles. Get a massage at least once a month during your training period and you'll feel a whole lot better in the process. You can use it as a reward for your hard work, and enjoy the numerous psychological and physiological benefits of massage.

Keep these things in mind and you'll put yourself in a position to stick to your training plan while avoiding injury along the way.

THE WEEK BEFORE, AND RACE DAY

Here are the things you need to remember the week before the race, and on the big day itself.

The week before: It's all about the preparation

A week before the race, you should be tapering. That means that you've cut your training mileage and focusing on getting ready for the race. At this point, it's perfectly natural to feel some jitters. You're excited, I get it; everyone is excited at this point in their lives.

Just don't let that excitement distract you from the ultimate goal. So what should you be doing a week before the race?

Taper

Technically, you should already be tapering 3 weeks before the race. Tapering begins as soon as you finished your longest training run and you're starting to cut back on your mileage. This period is designed to help your body recover from all the stresses of training so it can be at peak shape come race day.

The problem with many runners is that they often feel anxious during the taper period because they're not used to doing less just days before a race. We always want to be doing as much as we can to prepare and it seems weird that preparing for a race involves just sitting down on your ass and elevating your legs to rest.

The thing to remember during the taper period is to trust your training. You've put in the mileage. You've suffered through countless morning runs and you've put in all the work that is required.

The taper period is the time you give your body some rest. All that pounding would have taken its toll; during the taper period, you allow your body to heal and consolidate your training. During this time, all the damage would have to be repaired allowing you to be 100% on the day of the race.

So, what are the main attributes of a proper tapering that would allow you to be at your best on race day? Here are some guidelines:

Three weeks before the race

Reduce your weekly mileage to about 85% of your maximum. The training plans we attached already takes care of this period but it helps if you understand why you're seeing a drop-off in running volume after your longest run. The easiest way to do mileage reduction during the first taper week is to cut a day off of your training schedule; so, say, you run 5 days a week during your training, you can cut it to 4 days during your first taper week.

At the same time, make sure that you maintain your run intensity. Continue to run at your preferred pace while scaling the volume. This will allow your body to take less pounding but still maintain a high level of fitness.

Two weeks before the race

Continue cutting back on your mileage, this time up to 70% of maximum. If you've been doing 50 miles per week, you should be doing about 35 miles during this time. You should also eliminate your long runs and dedicate your weekend runs to "maintenance runs" which are basically short runs at target pace so keep your fitness up.

In terms of workout intensity, you should already avoid high intensity workouts at this period. At best, try one workout at medium intensity preferable very early in the week to give your body time to recover.

The week before the race

Here we go! You're almost there. Just one more week and you're already a marathon finisher.

During this week, reduce your mileage to about 20% of your maximum. This is basically a "rest week" with just a couple of runs at low intensity. If you need a quick jolt just to maintain confidence, try a short speed workout or fartlek at medium intensity so your legs know what it feels like to run at your preferred pace.

And that's it. Keep those things in mind in the days leading to the race and you'll feel a lot better about your chances of finishing strong.

Carboloading

Carboloading isn't an excuse for fat loading. Remember: you've trained hard and dropped weight. The last thing you need is gain all that weight back during the taper period leaving you sluggish and lethargic on race day. You want to fuel your performance engine but only enough for it to successfully complete the marathon. So, how do you do it?

As the name implies, it's all about loading carbs into your body. The end goal is to convert those carbs into glycogen stores in your muscles. The body burns both fat and glycogen during the run but the latter is a more efficient fuel that gets you from the start to the finish line in good spirits.

Running out of glycogen during the run leads to a phenomenon known as "hitting the wall." This happens when your body has to rely on fat for fuel; because fat burns much slower, you end up running slower in return.

As discussed in the previous chapter, your best option is to go for whole grain carbs. Rice is one good option but you can also go for other like bread, pancakes, bagels, waffle, tortillas and oatmeal. There are also plenty of fruits that provide a well-balance nutritional profile perfect for carboloading. This includes bananas, peers, peaches among others.

When carboloading, try to avoid high-fat foods like cheese, butter, oil, and even high protein foods. Fats and protein take a long time to be digested and they tend to make you feel bloated and heavy.

The mistake for most runners is the tendency to overeat during the last week heading to the marathon. Again, remember that you should make your diet work for you instead of sabotaging your nutrition and fitness. At the very least, think about the fact you're already reducing your training mileage at this time; by increasing your food intake significantly than normal, you're putting yourself in a perilous position. The likely outcome: a bigger, heavier you on race day! I'm sure you don't want that.

The best recommendation is to eat about 4 grams of carbs for every pound of body weight. One gram is roughly equal to 4 calories so if you're a 140-pound runner (63kg), you should look at a 2,240-calorie diet on a daily basis. In addition, you should also try to get up to 90% of your calories mainly from carbs so your body can efficiently pack fuel for the big day.

In terms of weight gain, it would be reasonable to expect a 4-pound (1.8kg) weight gain and that's okay. At that weight, you should still feel light enough while being able to successfully fuel for the race. Anything more than that and you have likely overeaten beyond what was necessary; anything less and you would have not eaten enough. This should give you a rough estimate of what you need to aim for during the carboloading period.

Lastly, you should consider carboloading only until 2 days before the race. Your body needs time to digest the food you have eaten and eating a heavy meal the day before can lead to serious bathroom issues on race day. A day before the race, you should already be eating light meals at more frequent intervals to allow your body to move the food out before you race.

Hydration

And then we come to hydration. While this is not a very complicated thing, you still need to think about it properly.

At the very least, try to get your body acclimatized to drinking the sports drinks that will be served on the day of the race. You should know this by just looking at the sponsors on the marathon ads. If not, you can always email the marathon secretariat to try and find out what they will be putting out on the course while you are racing.

The best hydration advice you can ever get is to drink plenty of fluids in the week leading up to the race. Don't worry about overhydrating. Your body cannot handle any excess water and will just pass it out naturally. The only thing you have to remember is to come into the race knowing that you are not dehydrated before you even started running. If you do that, then you're already doing all that you can to prepare your body for the challenge that lies at the end of the week.

Sleep

One thing that's not discussed in other marathon guides is the idea of sleep in the days leading up to the race. For fall marathon races in the US or Europe, this is often not an issue because the start-time isn't until mid-morning so you do not have to tweak your routine to adjust.

In tropical countries, however, many marathons start at 3 or 4 in the morning, and some even start at midnight. For this, you need to look at your sleep times and try to align your body clock to the race schedule.

The best suggestion is to use the week to gradually adjust your wake-up time. For example, if your race starts at 3AM on Sunday, start as early as Tuesday in adjusting your sleep habits. Sleep earlier and gradually try to wake up earlier too. If you normally wake up at 6AM, then move up your wake up time to 5AM on Wednesday, 4AM on Thursday, 3AM on Friday, and 2AM on Saturday to get you up to speed with your race wake-up time.

Of course, it is important to still get the right number of hours even if you wake up early so you need to adjust your sleeping time accordingly.

Preparing your race kit

The last thing you need to remember for the week before the race is to prepare everything that you need. You don't want to miss anything important as you race, and yet many have suffered from a sabotage race precisely because of minor things.

Here's a simple marathon checklist to help you get sorted with all your race needs.

Make sure you do this check a day or two before the race. It is recommended that you lay down everything that you need on the bed and pack them properly to make sure everything is accounted for. Remember: be deliberate. You want to be sure you have everything that you need so you don't get rattled or surprised on race day.

- [ ] Running Shoes
- [ ] Running Socks
- [ ] Singlet/Top
- [ ] Compression Shorts
- [ ] Jacket
- [ ] Jogging Pants
- [ ] Sports Bra (for women)
- [ ] Visor
- [ ] Extra Shirt
- [ ] Compression Sleeves
- [ ] Sunglasses
- [ ] Running Watch
- [ ] Heart Rate Monitor
- [ ] Bib Holder
- [ ] Gel Holder - Waistpack
- [ ] Slippers
- [ ] MP3 & Earphones
- [ ] Extra Underwear
- [ ] Extra Running Shoes

Miscellaneous preparation tips

Here are a few other miscellaneous reminders that you should check out before racing.

Clip your nails. Long toe nails will hurt at longer distances.

Apply petroleum jelly on race day to all body parts that are prone to chafing burns. Put it in your armpit, in the groin area, and between your toes. Also, try to carry a small petroleum jelly bottle with you during the race so if you need to re-apply along the way, you don't get caught empty handed.

Charge your gadgets. Running out of battery in the middle of the race can be a surprise factor that you don't want to deal with because it can knock you off your routine. Charge your phone, music player (if allowed), and running watch. Carry a spare battery pack if possible so you are prepared for any issue that can happen.

Of course, don't try and carry everything during the race. You're not going camping. Many of the things on the checklist are meant to keep your mind at ease or make you comfortable after the race. Leave them at the baggage area and only carry what you need. We'll cover this in more detail in the next section.

Try to get a bead on the weather on race so you can dress accordingly. Don't leave anything to chance. Make sure you have cold and warm weather clothes available so you can put on what's appropriate for the actual race condition.

Pay attention to these reminders so you don't encounter any surprises on the day of the race.

Race Day: Here we go!

So you've done the training, you're ready to race. The last thing that you need is to miss something that can turn your day from great to miserable.

Avoid all the potential problems and eliminate all the uncertainties with these race day suggestions.

Arrive early. This is perhaps the most important advice you will get for racing your first marathon. Many runners end up getting frazzled even before they cross the starting line because they come in late and then they have to rush through their preparations.

Don't allow yourself to be hurried because you no longer have the time

Your First Marathon

to do everything that you need. Come in early, at least an hour and a half before the race starts, so you have time to park your car, change into your racing outfit, scout the starting area for the best position, and get your warm-up done.

Don't try anything new on race day. We've already talked about this many times in the previous sections. You should have tried out your clothes, shoes, and even nutrition and hydration strategy during your long runs. Never ever do anything on race day that you wouldn't do on an ordinary training run or this can lead to issues that you may not be prepared to handle.

For breakfast, eat your usual pre-run meal. Don't try a bagel or peanut butter if you haven't eaten those before. You don't want to be running with an upset stomach a few kilometers into a 26 mile race.

If you fuel with energy bars or gels in your long runs, take one in 30 minutes before the start of the race. This is pre-fueling, and you need it to maximize your energy stores before you start out to run.

You should also drink a glass or two of sports drink but make sure you don't overhydrate. Overhdyrating is fine days before the race but not when you're minutes away from running the biggest race of your life. Just drink enough; too much will leave you feeling bloated and searching for the toilet 500 meters in.

Do some light warm-up before you run. Stretching depends from runner to runner; some runners do it, others don't. If you must have to, only stretch lightly so you don't pull a muscle before you even started.

You should also do some light running to warm up your leg muscles. Short 400-meter jogs to get your body up to temperature is a great way to start any race.

Lineup with runners that are more or less your speed. You don't want to line-up with the fast runners or you'll be suckered into running very fast out of the gate. You also don't want to be stuck at the back because you'll have to weave through hundreds of slower runners to get to the front and that consumes a lot of energy.

Find your crowd and line-up accordingly so you can maintain a stable pace right out of the gate.

Be conservative with your early race pacing. It's tempting to run out fast: but don't or you'll burn yourself quickly.

Start out at a slightly slower pace than your target to allow your body to fully warm-up. Once you're a mile into the race, you can judge your condition and adjust your pace accordingly.

Hydrate and eat according to your training routine. You should have already practiced this by now. The rule is to drink 5-8 ounces (142-227ml) of liquid every 15 minutes. You can adjust this depending on the placement of water stations along the course. The one thing you have to remember is to never wait to feel thirst before drinking. Thirst is already a late signal for dehydration. Drink ahead, but not too much, to keep your body fluids at a stable level throughout the race.

If you feel any discomfort in the middle of the run, try to walk it off or stretch it. This will often come up around 22 miles in when your legs have taken some level of pounding. It's alright to stretch and loosen your muscles to avoid cramping so don't feel obligated to push always. Listen to your body and race accordingly.

If possible, find a runner that's running at the same pace as you and run together. The marathon is an individual sport but you can help and be helped by others. It is so much more comforting to have somebody to run with through all the miles that you still need to cover so find a runner that shares this idea and power through together. Remember: you do not have to speak to each other if you don't want to, but just having someone run beside you can be very uplifting and motivating.

Have fun! You're doing this because it's fun. Enjoy the scenery, the crowd, the sight of other runners on the road. Make it an experience you will never forget – for the right reasons – and you'll cross the finish line happier than if you treated the whole race as a chore.

Smile. Photographers will be out on the course for the official marathon photos. Smile and hold your pose so you'll have great pictures to remind you of the fun that you've had as you raced! Congratulations on completing your marathon journey!

May this be the first of many more, and may it be a story that you can share to many others to inspire them to take up running. It may have been demanding, yes, but the reward of conquering your dreams will never be matched.

So enjoy and soak in the glory of becoming a marathon finisher, because you certainly deserve it!

Marathon Recovery

You might have finished your marathon but your job still isn't done. If you want to quickly bounce back and not suffer through the agonizing post-marathon leg pains that you'll find on YouTube, you have to be proactive with your recovery plan.

Here are some tips to help you recover as quickly as possible in the time for the next marathon.

You need to focus on re-fueling your body after it has depleted all of its stores. Bananas, energy bars, and sports drinks – even fruits if those are available – can help you quickly load up on carbs and protein. A light meal after a good race is certainly something that you should consider planning ahead for.

You should also find time to change into something more comfortable. Get a jacket if you're feeling cold, or change your shirt if you can. Slip into some comfortable slippers to allow your feet to rest.

Once you get back home or into your hotel room, consider an ice batch just as you would do R.I.C.E. after a training run. After an ice batch, consider a quick nap or a walk-around to loosen your legs and flush out the lactic acid. That will reduce the likelihood of muscle soreness and will allow you to walk upright the following day. Using compression clothes is also a great way to speed up recovery after the race.

As for running, try not to get back on the road for the next three days. Get a hot tub soak and some light stretching every few hours, and always focus on proper nutrition to supply your body with all the nutrients it needs to repair damaged muscles.

From day 4 to 7, you can consider one short run for 2 to 3 miles at a very easy pace just to quickly get back into the thick of things. Still focus on nutrition and hydration.

During the second week, you can probably get in 2 to 3 more days of running for no more than 3 miles and still at an easy pace. Cross-training with a bike or a swim is also a great way to get your muscles engaged again.

If you do all these correctly, you should be back into proper form within 3 weeks and ready to take on a new challenge. Perhaps, it's now time to plan for your second marathon?

CONCLUSION

The marathon is a great personal achievement, but it also entails a lot of personal sacrifice, some planning, and definitely a lot of commitment and hours.

Still, you don't need to go blind into the process. This book is designed to help guide you through each harrowing step so you can identify all the potential danger areas and plan accordingly.

Remember, the secret to succeeding in the marathon is planning, and the determination to stick to your training plan if your health allows for it. Always be cautious of your training runs, but also take time to listen to your body to eliminate the risk of injuries.

I hope I was able to successfully guide you through your first marathon.

I wish you many more, and I hope to see you on the road in one of these future races.

Made in the USA
Lexington, KY
30 December 2015